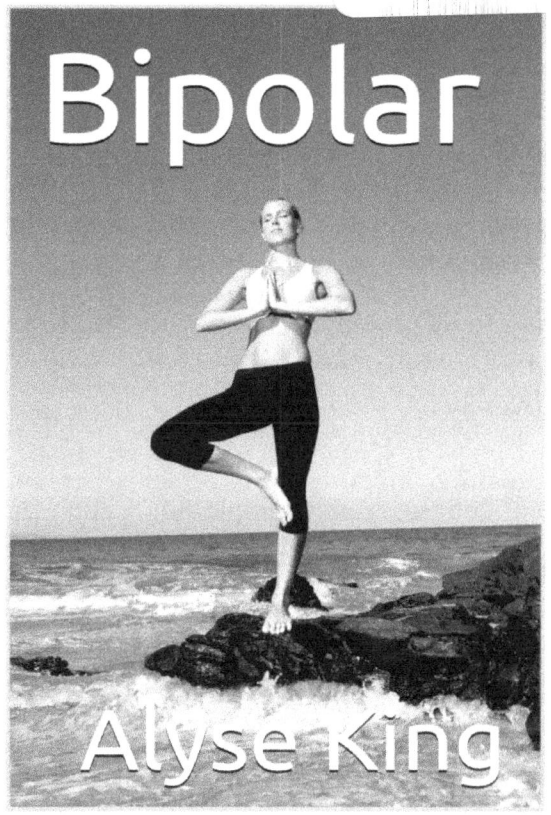

Alyse King

... "When sickness will be no more."
Rev 21:3-4

DEDICATION

I dedicate this book to my precious daughter for her strength, courage, and endurance during her most difficult years

"A heart broken and crushed, O God you will not despise," Psalm 51:17 (NWT)

Preface

Parents all over the world who care about their children's mental health will want to read this book. I was shocked when bipolar struck my youngest daughter. She was 16 years old.

Once I received that devastating diagnosis, I devoted all my waking hours to caring for her. I worked tirelessly until I received successful results.

Like any other illness, knowledge and early detection of bipolar disorder is vitally important to prevent years of pain and hardships. Unfortunately, the symptoms during the early stages were truly deceptive and confusing. They were unsuspecting and gradual, which made it impossible to detect them as the beginning signs of mental illness, or differentiate them from those turbulent teenage years.

The book provides an overview of my experience as the medical conditions with my daughter developed. It details her coping and recovery process. It also provides useful information along with references for further information about bipolar disorders.

It is impossible to imagine a journey into a life with bipolar disorders. It is a journey happening to someone else's sons and daughters. It is a journey that is, at times, embarrassing to tell. It is a journey that is all too heart breaking. At times, I felt that death would have been more comforting than living with the struggles and heartbreaks of seeing my daughter in turmoil day after day.

Immediately after receiving the diagnosis, I researched everything that I could find about bipolar. I pulled out old magazines and books. I started reading and learning everything I could find. I went to the public library, and did research. I then cross-referenced all my research materials to ensure I had correct, accurate and current information for myself and to convey to my daughter.

For years, with the severity and the debilitation from this illness, there was a near zero chance that my daughter would lead a normal life again.

Her inability to accomplish any of life's tasks caused the many distresses, resulting in further low self-esteem and self-worth.

She desperately needed to cope, as the fears of bipolar were greater than her coping abilities. It was a very weighty and challenging task, but I continued without let up to find new and different ways to help her. Learning new ways to cope was an on-going process for us.

It was important never push her or criticize her, but allow her to make progress with my support. I let her learn at her own pace, in her own way, and in her own time. At times when she needed her own space, I gave her space when she wanted to be alone.

Life with Bipolar was and still is a harrowing experience for my daughter. It required my patience, perseverance and all my love and support for her.

I accepted my daughter's mental illness, not as failures, but as limitations. Even though my core purpose in life as a mother was to nurture her, when she became ill, my mission was to help her to cope, and heal while learning to live with her limitations.

This is a book of not giving up. All the recommendations offered in this book helped my daughter on her difficult road to recovery.

Introduction

This journey gives a panoramic view of the struggles with bipolar disorder. This is a compelling story of strength, courage, resilience and hope. It describes in detail how my daughter coped with this horrible disorder.

What inspired me and kept me driven to share this, was the unforgettable, painful journey and the grim prognosis. FINALLY, THERE WAS HOPE OF RECOVERY.

The objective of the book is to increase the awareness of families and caregivers. This book gives an overview of how to recognize some of the emerging warning signs of bipolar.

The reader has an advantaged point of view as she takes you through a journey of hopelessness to the joyous moment that begins the recovery process. This book is intended to assure other families that there is hope of recovery.

It includes some of the coping skills that helped my daughter recover from severe bipolar.

My Daughter's Journey

This journey began on another beautiful, starry night in Southern California. My daughter was upstairs alone. I was home and enjoying the evening with the family and playing with my first grandchild when she began to have a serious bipolar breakdown.

Imagine the scene that night when I realized that she was breaking down. She was in anguish. Her sisters were in anguish. I was in anguish. Once again, we experienced another harrowing account of the subtleness, deceptiveness and destructiveness of mental illness.

Prior to this time, she had already showed signs of serious turbulences happening to her. She had already begun to isolate herself in her room. She was angry all the time. She was depressed. She was despondent. She was distraught. She had trouble going to school No one else noticed these symptoms even though I tried to get help.

Once a quiet, well behaved girl, she now became more withdrawn, and isolated herself in her bedroom for weeks at a time. Those weeks turned into months.

The months leading up to the night she broke down were difficult for her. Most days she was not feeling good. She had been complaining about having severe headaches. I took her to the doctor several times. The doctors could not find what was causing her headaches.

As usual, she was alone upstairs in her bedroom, and I was downstairs with the rest of the family. My daughter came downstairs in distress, much more than usual. I knew that something was seriously wrong. She was holding her head and crying. She looked frightened. I started to worry.

She looked at me and in an urgent voice, said, *"Mom can you come up stairs, please?"* I immediately handed my granddaughter to her dad and followed her upstairs. She anxiously kept repeating, *"Mom I don't know what is wrong with me, something is happening to me."*

Instantly, I was in agony. I cried out to God for help. It was too familiar a scene. *"This can't be happening again."*

I don't remember if I felt like I just wanted to die instead of seeing my child suffering. Whatever my feelings were, they were feelings of trauma.

I already knew what was happening to my daughter. That thought shook me to my core, and I began to tremble. Imagine the pain I felt in seeing another one of my children having a psychotic breakdown. I started to weep. Between my tears, I comforted her and told her, *"that it was ok to feel afraid, and that she would feel better soon."*

I dreaded this because I knew too well the hardships that were ahead and I knew I needed strength more than ever to cope with it. Like the countless times before, I started to pray. I had full faith that my prayers would once again give me the strength and courage to endure another tragedy with another child.

It was another heartrending journey. The uncertainties of how my daughter would accept her illness worried me. ***"How can this happen to my daughter?" "Where did I go wrong a second time?" "Am I at fault?"*** These were all the thoughts going through my mind. **I wished that I could spare her from the hardships ahead.**

I immediately began hugging my daughter and kept reassuring her, *"I love you and you will be ok." "You will be ok."*

I called out for my other two daughters. They rushed into the bedroom began comforting her and kept telling her they loved her. She could not be comforted. Her two sisters were frightened; they were visibly shaking, sad and bewildered. This was also a difficult, tear-jerking journey for them.

"I must act quickly." I kept thinking to myself. I wasted no time. In haste, her two sisters and I rushed her to the emergency room, all the while comforting her and calling out to God to give us courage and strength.

The hospital paged the on-call psychiatrist since none was on duty that night. In the meantime, my daughter kept panicking. All we could do was comfort her and continue to reassure her of our love.

As the minutes became hours, we became restless and could no longer sit still. We started pacing back and forth. The stress was affecting all of us. We did not talk to each other. As we waited, we were consumed with our own private thoughts.

Before long, I started to feel angry, and kept thinking, *'Why is this happening again?'*

It seemed to take an eternity for the psychiatrist to arrive. My daughter continued to be frantic. Finally, he arrived. He evaluated her, prescribed medications and referred her to the county mental health facility for follow-up treatments.

It was now past midnight and I found a pharmacy that was still open. My daughter immediately started taking the medications. Unfortunately, they were not the proper ones. They did not help her. The doctor had prescribed medicines for anxiety. They were not the right ones for her condition.

We followed up at the county mental health clinic. The psychiatrist at the clinic prescribed mood stabilizers as well as medication for psychosis. This time the medications begun to stabilized her – somewhat.

After a few more visits, the treating psychiatrist *diagnosed her as having Psychosis with Major Depression!* ***"OH MY GOD, NOT AGAIN!"*** I yelled out.

Many years later, after a through re-evaluation, she was *re-diagnosed as having Bipolar Disorder*.

I knew that bi-polar disorder was a difficult and serious disease, one that could ruin her life. Being armed with this knowledge enabled me to work extremely hard to care for her.

A piercing pain was ripping through my heart. I was very heartbroken. "How could any one family survive this second devastating tragedy?" I kept thinking to myself.

My strong faith ***and previous experiences*** played a vital role in my survival of this unbearable journey.

During the months before her break down, I was still reeling from my son's first psychotic breakdown. I was also still dealing with many struggles and challenges at home as well as my own stresses and depression. The years that led up to my daughter's breakdown, were tumultuous and very similar to my son's pre-psychotic experiences.

She too was depressed and isolated herself. She expressed anger and rage towards me. She had severe delusions of grandeur. For months, she was convinced that she was the image of a popular, **'TV soap opera actress**.' She even imitated her hairstyles. For my daughter, it was real. **For me it was painful.**

Although I could identify a few of my daughter's symptoms such as depression, isolation, and the extreme emotional mood swings, it was unthinkable that mental illness would strike another child, so harshly and viciously.

Although both the elementary and middle school years were manageable for her because she was a bright student, she too had a difficult and challenging time attending high school.

During her first year in high school, she began having severe headaches. At least, that was how she described them. I took her to the doctor. After a thorough examination, he could not find anything that was causing her headaches.

Previously, my daughter was fitted with braces and retainers. I took her back to the Orthodontist to determine whether that could be the cause of her headaches. The Orthodontist assured me that being fitted for or wearing braces and retainers would not have caused headaches.

In retrospect, the symptoms were not headaches; rather, my daughter was experiencing psychosis. She became more erratic, irrational and filled with anger. Eventually, she could not cope with school. That led to me asking the school for help.

After the school psychologist met with my daughter, she told me that she could not find anything wrong with her.

That was an absolute misdiagnosis!
My daughter was seriously ill.

At times, even trained professionals, such as school psychologists and Interns with years of experience, cannot detect warning signs of mental illness.

This was the second time that trained professionals failed my children.

Coping with this illness was difficult for her. She eventually dropped out of high school. She later enrolled in Alternative Education. That too overwhelmed her. I was devastated and heartbroken, again.

As the months slowly dragged by, she became more agitated, aggressive and reclusive. Her symptoms continued and worsened.

Shortly after the night of her psychotic episode, she began antipsychotic treatments that prevented hospitalization. During this period, she tried taking a host of other medications. Although there were slight improvements, she suffered many side effects.

While taking the antipsychotic drug, Zyphrexia, she gained a massive amount of weight. She was less than100 pounds before taking the drug, and after taking this medication, she ballooned to almost 200 pounds within a 2-year period. She was extremely saddened by this and her emotional state worsened.

As time dragged on, she became more and more despondent about her weight. She asked her psychiatrist, on several occasions, to discontinue Zyphrexia. **The doctor refused and she kept taking it!**

To our greatest surprise, during one of her doctor's visits, the **psychiatrist told her to eat carrot sticks to lose the weight! We were shocked.** She never returned to that psychiatrist.

We knew that Zyphrexia was the cause of the weight gain.

My daughter was very despondent on a daily basis. I comforted her as much as possible.

Soon after, I found another doctor that prescribed new medications that did not cause my daughter to gain weight, but she continued to struggle to find effective medications that would stabilize the bi-polar disorders.

After many years of struggles and relapses, excellent medications were prescribed and they are effectively controlling her illness.

It was with quick thinking getting her to the hospital, obtaining the proper medications and the family's love and support that helped her through her horrible ordeals. She is now progressing well and experiencing success in her daily life.

Although there were many challenges for her to overcome during her coping and recovery journey, she has risen to those challenges. She is continuing to progress well and finding real purpose in her life.

No Cure

In reality, no scientific research has resulted in findings to support a possible cure for bipolar. However, thanks to modern, effective and available medicines the intensity and frequency of the illness are manageable. While the illness continues to cause minor impairments in function despite treatments and family support, my family and I successfully live with this illness.

If bipolar is untreated, or if not treated in a timely manner, the frightening reality of suicide is a possibility. The quicker one begins the right treatment program, the better the chance of recovery will be.

If my daughter's bipolar were left untreated, it would have completely ruined her life. Even with treatments with medications and therapy, her condition was severely affected. Her development into womanhood, her educational goals and having a fulfilling and productive life had diminished.

It has been stated that approximately 20% of children and adolescents experience mental disorders. Half of all mental illnesses begin by the age of 14.

"More than 90% of all cases of suicide are associated with mental disorders such as depression, schizophrenia, and alcoholism," notes Dr. Benedetto Saraceno, Director of the Department of Mental Health for WHO.

What is Bipolar Disorder

"Bipolar typically consists of both manic and depressive episodes separated by period of normal mood. Manic episodes involve elevated or irritable mood, over-activity, pressure of speech, inflated self-esteem and a decreased need for sleep. People who have manic attacks but do not experience depressive episodes are also classified as having bipolar disorder," stated the World Health Organization.

"Bipolar affective disorder – This disorder affects about 60 million people worldwide. It typically consists of both manic and depressive episodes separated by periods of normal mood. Manic episodes involve elevated or irritable mood, over-activity, …. Decreased need for sleep, inflated self-esteem," stated the World Health Organization 2014.

It has been stated that bipolar may affect approximately 2 percent of the American population.

People who have manic attacks but do not experience depressive episodes are also classified as having bipolar disorder.

It has been stated that immediate family members are 8-18 times likely to develop this illness. Having a family member or members with bipolar, may make other family members more likely to suffer with major depression, like I did when I cared for my children.

It has been stated that bipolar affects both men and women equally and normal begins in young adulthood.

Warning Signs I Missed

Prior to the diagnosis, there were months and years that bipolar traumatized the family.

My daughter's young life was already derailing. A turbulent life had already begun for her and my family. Gone were the happy days. Gone was my daughter's pleasant, happy very short life.

The anger I felt because I missed those subtle warning signs of mental illness were also unimaginable as was the pain and sadness that over powered me.

A few years prior to her breakdown, she started to show many troubling signs of emotional disturbances. She was in a state of euphoria with unusually high energy. Her thoughts were racing continuously.

She was not able to explain why he felt a particular way, or why she uttered certain statements. Her behavior was difficult to manage. She refused to cooperate with the family. She was never happy. I kept wondering why my daughter was behaving in this rebellious manner. It was uncharacteristic of her to behave this way. She - like my son had always been an obedient child when she was growing up, now she is an out-of-control adolescent.

As time went on, a host of other symptoms began to emerge. She could no longer control her anger. She was very easily frustrated.

As time went on, her symptoms worsened. She eventually dropped out of Alternative Education.

She lived a life in complete torment.

I kept encouraging her not to give up and reassuring her that she - would in time - have a better, brighter future because I knew she could. However, the symptoms continued.

Like my son, her educational and career dreams vanished in front of my eyes. Again, I was very heart broken at the thought that she must feel devastated at realizing that her life had fallen apart – because of an illness.

She kept retreated from everyone and locked herself in her room. Her bedroom became her haven. She continued to be distraught, distressed, depressed and despondent. She continued to be anxious and frustrated. It was extremely difficult to interact with her. She continued to be angry, aggressive and restless. She continued to be irrational and erratic. These symptoms continued to interfere with her ability to function.

During this entire time, my daughter never complained. Yes, I was happy that she frequently discussed her feelings with me. She tried to be so courageous, so strong, and so brave!

As months turned into years, the symptoms worsened. She did not care about anything or anyone. Her outlook for the future was pessimistic. She lost her self-esteem and self-confidence. She did not socialize with anyone.

As time went on, she became more hostile towards me and constantly screamed at me. There were tensions and anger. Her sleeping pattern became more erratic. One moment she was irrational and verbally abusive, the next moment she was calm and – oh, so sweet to be with.

When she was in the manic stages, she could not sleep and was up all night long. During this period ideas flowed through her mind and she would come up with many creative business ideas. When she was in the depressive stages, she was practically bed-ridden.

After experiencing all those symptoms, I did not know they were signs of the onset of bipolar.

Bipolar - like schizophrenia is also one of the worst of all mental illnesses and once again, I missed all the warning signs because I could not imagine mental illness was strike another one of my children!

As a parent, I have had many regrets and have made many mistakes while raising my children. But my biggest mistake was my **ignorance.** I knew something serious was happening to her but truly thought those symptoms were just difficulties associated with teenage years, 'acting out,' as the experts say. I just thought her behaviors were unacceptable, not realizing that perhaps my daughter was experiencing psychosis. Unfortunately, they were much more than teenage difficulties. My daughter was, in fact, very chronically ill.

HOW IT PAINED MY HEART FOR MISSING ALL THOSE SYMPTOMS!

It has been stated that approximately 20% of children and adolescents experience mental disorders. Half of all mental illnesses begin by the age of 14. If untreated, these conditions severely influence children's development, their educational attainments and their potential to live fulfilling and productive lives.

I felt that I failed my daughter. I felt ashamed. I was heart-broken and had many regrets for years.

Warning Signs

There are countless warning signs. Becoming aware of them will ensure that mental illness is diagnosed early. Some of my daughter's warning signs of bipolar include:

In the past bipolar disorder was called manic depression. With bipolar, my daughter experienced prolonged episodes of manias, also known as intense hyperactivity or depressions also known as experiencing devastating low periods.

- Decreasing ability to function.
- Inability to begin a task or to complete a task.
- Acting out of character.
- Quitting school.
- Ceasing to work.
- Talking about violence, threatening comments, or talking about suicide or hurting someone.
- Isolating oneself from family and friends.
- Manic periods and depressed periods.
- Acting quickly.

- Lacking focus and concentration.
- Distorting reality.
- Moodiness.
- Failing to comply with instructions, and rules.
- Refusing to see a doctor or take medications.
- Loss weight/gain weight
- Manipulating everyone.
- Arguing.
- No appetite.
- Disturbed sleep.
- Forgetting, imaging and recalling imaginary details as information.
- Poorly executing instructions.
- Uncommunicative.
- Inability to read or reflect.
- No interest in finding pleasure in anything.

Acknowledging bipolar as a serious sickness rather than a "troubled person," "problem person," "difficult person," will help us focus on how we can support our loved one.

It has been stated that people with bipolar mood disorders have high mortality rates ranging from

35% higher to twice as high as the general population.

Support Group

My daughter did not attend support groups. There were very few available in those days and hard to find. Years earlier while my son was hospitalized, I needed support. I contacted the local National Association of Mental Health (NAMI) for resources. They recommended that I attend a group session in one of the local hospitals. I recalled how shocking my first visit was. There were many distraught; elderly parents there discussing the challenges and obstacles they were experiencing with their mentally ill, adult sons and daughters. I did not want to be in that position.

I did not think this group was able to help me. I began working with my son and daughter at home.

Counseling Sessions

As the months became years, gone were the days of calm, peace, happiness, laughter and enjoyment from my home. They were replaced with complete chaos. There were immense hardships, distresses and depravation that we had never before experienced. My daughter's counseling sessions did help her somewhat. She still sees a therapist from time to time. She keeps in mind that an imbalance of the brain chemistry cannot be reasoned away with logic overnight. It has been taking years with much patience.

Health Care Professionals

For almost two decades, many health care professionals treated my daughter. During that entire period, no one has ever recommended a book, magazine, article or any other reading material that could have helped with the coping and recovery process.

Health Insurance

Health care is a basic human need. It is equally as necessary and important as food, clothing and shelter. No matter who we are, or our economic and social status, we all need health care. While many today are suffering from the lack of adequate mental health care, I am very appreciative that my daughter received quality health care during much of the time that she was grappling with her mental illness.

Inadequate mental health insurance or the lack of mental health insurance is a very risky situation for society. Having adequate mental health insurance is crucial for the prevention of relapses, and suicide. Additionally, this ensures that they do not harm themselves, family or community members.

During the untreated periods of bipolar, suicide is a possibility. Once a person obtain the right medications and maintained a daily intake regimen, those feelings stopped. It is just good common sense for everyone to have access to mental health treatments.

Friends & Relatives

Both my son and daughter faced many challenges with isolation, discrimination and stigmas.

My daughter's old friends are long gone. New friends are hard to find. Relatives still ignores her. Some still do not bother to ask how she is doing.

Today, my daughter is able to handle those rejections. They both know that those who turned their backs on them were, and probably still are, ignorant about mental illness.

Why not be the first to show kindness and concern to someone with mental illness. Perhaps, try to put yourself in the ill person's place, and try to visualize how you would want to be treated. Offer a listening ear, or extend a helping hand, just show you care.

Oh! How refreshing it felt when my children are greeted with kind words.

Medication and Side Effects

"Effective treatments are available for the treatment of the acute phase of bipolar disorder and the prevention of relapse. These medicines stabilize mood. Psychosocial support is an important component of treatment." (WHO.)

It has been stated that, 'there are effective strategies for preventing mental disorders such as depression and bipolar. There are effective treatments for mental disorders and ways to alleviate the suffering caused by them.'

For over 16 years, several psychiatrists treated my daughter. They treated bipolar with a host of different medications. Most of them were ineffective for her condition. During her first psychotic breakdown, the psychiatrist initially treated her with antipsychotic drugs. For a long time that were ineffective. Her symptoms continued. When the proper medication is prescribed for her she can live a somewhat, "normal," life.

Mood stabilizers are the primary treatment for the maintenance treatment of bipolar disorder. Lithium for example stabilizes mood.

An aggressive medication regime was needed to avoid going to the psychiatric ward.

Along with medications, psychosocial support is a necessary part of her treatment program. Even though they do help her, it is a constant daily struggles for her.

Her primary side effect from taking the medications was weight gain – and it still is.

Isolation

Loneliness is one of the factors that lead people to depression and suicide. My daughter's tendency was to isolate herself. I had to make myself available to ensure that – that she does not isolate herself for long periods. During these periods, negative thoughts creep up and she begins to get lonely.

"Children with mental disorders face major challenges with stigma, isolation and discrimination, as well as lack of access to health care and educational facilities," (WHO).

Loneliness

It has been stated that loneliness is one of the factors that lead people to depression and suicide. In order for my daughter to cope and function, continuous support from family and friends is crucial for her. Negative thoughts plagued her when she is alone.

It has been stated that a great number of those who had committed suicide, everyday life was lonely. They have lots of spare time but few social contacts."

Remissions

During remission, our lives returned to normal. It was a pleasant time in the family. My daughter felt a sense of belonging and felt good about herself. We enjoyed a 'normal' life. We engaged in fun activities and enjoyed each other's companionship. We laughed, and laughed and laughed. Throughout this entire ordeal, my daughter managed to retain her sense of humor. She did daily chores such as preparing her meals, washing her dishes, shopping and doing her laundry. The remission days are stress free, anxiety free, and depression free.

How My Daughter Coped

As mental illness rocked my world, and terror reigned over my family, it devastated us. The storminess of mental illness exhausted me, and my family fell to pieces. The most agonizing part of all was that it might never end. Yet, I set aside my anxieties and fears and courageously calmed my children's fears.

My daughter's illness did not present overnight; she suffered years of gradual break down. At times, the symptoms were frequent and severe. Other times, they were less severe and less frequent.

My daughter's erratic behavior from bipolar disorder was a constant source of grief and confusion to the family. One moment she was happy and laughing and in an instant, she went in a state of withdrawal, despondent and then went into isolation. This would last for days and weeks at a time. It was a time of great confusion and struggle for her and the family.

And, for those 16 years, my family lived with doubts and fears. The challenges seemed insurmountable.

There was no stability in her life, but her resilient spirit was outstanding.

For almost all of those years, my daughter complied with instruction to take her medications.

Mental illnesses took my daughter on a vicious emotional rollercoaster journey that was beyond my wildest imagination. This journey changed her life in drastic ways. This journey was long and arduous. Navigating them throughout those years was a trek during a dark, stormy, unending night.

I cannot accurately describe the torment that she suffered from living with bipolar.

During her depressed stage, she was more prone to thoughts of suicide. During her manic stage, she lacked the understanding of what was wrong from right.

During this period, she agonized because she was not able to enjoy her teenage years and relationships or look forward to the joys of marriage and parenthood. Bipolar robbed her of her happiness and joy of life.

How well my daughter cope with her illnesses would depend on her own positive outlook of the future, and leaving her losses and all regrets behind her.

With the proper medications, therapy, an exercise program, I began helping my daughter to develop coping skills with a sense of urgency. Since I didn't have any formal mental illness education or training, it was difficult to help her learn to cope. However, I was able to share with her *everything I learned* from research about her illness. I also shared with her the knowledge I gained while caring for my son as well as my accumulated years of working experiences.

Humor

Humor played an integral role in the recovery process. My daughter and I spent countless hours in silly laughter. We behaved as if we were two children having a lot of fun. During the first 16 years of her illness, my daughter and I spent a vast amount of hours talking about silly, trifling *many of which made no sense at all, but were very funny. We would tell each other that we were going on a laughing trip*, and then we would both burst out laughing much harder. No sooner did we stop laughing, sometimes only for a moment, before we would look at each other and burst out laughing again. We would tell each other that if someone heard us, they would think we were both going crazy.

For over two decades, many of my relatives referred to me as, "crazy." No, I was not crazy. I just wanted to keep my mind healthy. Humor and laughter helped us.

Today, my daughter continues to use laughter as therapy, and it is still extremely successful. Those little, nonsensical exchanges and behaviors were the very activities that helped my daughter to begin walking on her road to recovery.

Some Common Sense Steps

I began training my son and daughter by using *practical, common sense steps*, as follows:

SURPASSING LOVE

Like all children, my son and daughter flourished on my complete love and nurturing of them.

EMOTIONAL SUPPORT

They coped by accepting the emotional support I provided. I was by their side when they were fearful, when they were lonely or when they were just feeling sad. I comforted them. They needed to feel hopeful instead of experiencing feelings of failure and disappointment. I found ways to commend and encourage them.

CLEAR IDEA

I wanted them to have a clear idea of their illnesses and the skills I believed would help them to heal the fastest.

ACCEPTANCE

For the first several years, because of the *severity* of their illnesses, compounded with their complete denial of their mental illnesses, it was impossible for them to advance to the acceptance stage. I used the compare between millions of people suffering from physical illnesses such as heart disease, stroke, cancer or diabetes, who must accept their illnesses, and the millions of others who are struggling with depression, stresses, or experiencing psychosis. Both groups must accept their illnesses before they will begin to heal.

BALANCE

I taught them how to have a balanced view of their illnesses and treat them the same as any other illnesses.

BELIEVE

I wanted desperately for them to believe that they would recover. Once they believed in themselves and trusted in their beliefs, they began walking down their pathways to recovery.

First, they started coping. Then, they began advancing toward recovery.

ONE STEP

I encouraged them by telling them to take one small step at a time because each step was necessary for them to make small changes in their lives.

SMALL CHANGES

I taught them how to make small changes. They eventually understood that the only way to begin changing was by accepting their illnesses. After many years, they finally understood that no matter how small the changes in their thinking and lives were, those changes were vitally important to accepting their illnesses and helping them to cope.

HOPE

They quickly learned to embrace hope. They held on to the hope of recovery. They never gave up of hoping for recovery.

ASHAMED

In the beginning, they were ashamed to tell anyone that they were mentally ill. Over time, they were able to overcome their shame by realizing that there were no reasons to feel ashamed of their mental illness because it may suddenly strike anyone at any time.

HUMILIATED

At first, they felt humiliated by their mental illnesses. I engrained in them the fact that they did not need to feel ashamed. As the years passed, they ignored any feelings of humiliation and ignored anyone who tried to humiliate them.

SUFFERINGS

In time, they understood that they were not the only ones who are suffering, and that millions of others around the world were suffering from a form of mental illness. They also understood that those who are currently unaffected might someday succumb to mental illness.

FAULT

In the beginning, they felt that they might have caused their illnesses. Gratefully, they coped well when they understood that mental illness was not their fault, they did not cause it.

ANXIETY

They had periods when they suffered great anxieties, but I encouraged them to live by the scriptures encouragement not to worry about the future because tomorrow will have its own anxieties, problems, challenges and difficulties.

COURAGE

Happily, they did not allow the bitter effects of their illnesses to rob them of their courage to continue their lives.

NEVER GAVE UP

My daughter never gave up in their fight to survive their illnesses. They never gave in and never gave out either.

LOOKED BACK

I encouraged them to never look back on their past because there was nothing there to see. As a result, they seldom wondered what their lives might have been.

HOME ENVIRONMENT

They coped best when our home environment was supportive, compassionate and peaceful. They felt safe and unafraid.

GOOD DAYS

They distinguished their good days from their bad days. They appreciated and enjoyed the good days and did not waste time worrying about the other days when they were not feeling very well, or when their minds were deteriorating.

DISCERNMENT

They knew their limits and exited situations that could emotionally stress them.

REASSURANCE

When they felt depressed, I reassured them and reminded them, that their situation would improve.

FAILURES

They had many feelings of failure, but they learned to accept them and used them as motivational tools for their healing.

NEGATIVITY

They coped well when they ignored negativity. They recognized negativity in all its forms, extricated themselves from those situations and dwelled on positive thoughts and displaying positive traits. They also excelled when I did not accentuate their negative traits.

ENCOURAGEMENT

They thrived and coped well when others and I encouraged as well as reassured them with kind, comforting words. They felt refreshed.

APPRECIATE

When anyone showed genuine interest, offered sincere words of commendation or reassured them with a smile, they appreciated it.

KIND WORDS

Kind words from others were refreshing. They have power and they helped in the healing process.

PHONE CALLS

They appreciated any friends or relatives who called to check on them or to say hello.

VISITOR

They especially appreciated when anyone visited them.

SOCIAL SKILLS

I taught them social skills. They visited friends and relatives who were kind, comforting, encouraging, understanding, positive, supportive and sympathetic. When friends greeted them warmly and with kind words, as well as listened to them, they progressed.

SUPPORT

They learned to accept any genuine offer of support from family and friends, and it was extremely refreshing when family and friends showed interest in them. In contrast, they avoided everyone who was critical and judgmental, including relatives who accused them of being 'lazy.'

RELAPSES

As time went on, they coped well when they understood how important it was to prevent any relapses, once they appreciated that frequent relapses significantly reduced their chances of recovery, they eagerly cooperated with the doctors' instructions and my retraining efforts.

PERSONAL SKILLS

They coped well when they developed personal skills for daily living with such activities as maintaining personal hygiene and etiquette.

HOME SKILLS

Years into their illnesses, as their health improved, they developed self-reliance skills such as performing light, household chores; doing their laundry; cleaning their rooms; washing their dishes; and preparing light meals.

ROUTINE

They had a daily routine such as taking the prescribed dosage of medication at the designated frequency.

MONEY SKILLS

Later, as they both progressed, they acquired advanced skills, such as money management. At first, although money had little value to them, I gave them an allowance to splurge on comfort food such as pizza, favorite smoothies and burgers.

I BEGAN TEACHING THEM TO REBUILD THEMSELVES BY DEVELOPING THEIR SKILLS AND TALENTS.

SELF: I helped them rebuild their self-worth and self-confidence to enable them to look forward to re-entering the workforce.

ENVISION: They coped by clearly envisioning what physical comforts they wanted and who they wanted to become.

FOCUS: They visualized their lives as completely free from illnesses. They did not focus on their illnesses. Instead, they focused on their talents, skills and abilities.

ADHERENCE: I was adamant about their strict adherence to medical appointments, and following prescribed instructions.

DECISIONS: They made independent decisions and learned appropriate, decisive self-expression.

THRIVE: They thrived when they knew that they were cared for, understood and appreciated regardless of their mentally challenged status.

OPTIMISM: In spite of all those struggles, my son and daughter displayed an incredible amount of zeal and optimism for their future life. As bleak as the outlook may have been, they were optimistic.

VISUALIZED*:* They both visualized a positive, hopeful future.

POSITIVE: They remained positive throughout their journeys that they would learn to cope and that they would recover.

EMPOWERMENT: My children's lives were in total upheaval much of the time because of the changing tides of mental illness. Not just from day to day, but in many instances, from hour to hour. For them to cope, with any degree of success, meant that they had to *be constantly uplifted, and encouraged* as well as informed about any new treatments and medications. I empowered them by reading uplifting verses to them from the bible's book of Psalms and Proverbs. Their spirits were uplifted.

GOALS: After their symptoms decreased, I established goals. They were small goals that were reachable and attainable.

PLAN OF ACTION

I continued to assist them in their plans for the future. I instituted a well thought out Plan of Action that included the furthering of their education, developing pre-job training skills, job search skills and work force participation skills.

SPIRITUALITY

Above all else, they consciously invested in their personal spiritual development as well as laid a faith-based foundation, which ensured that they developed the strength to successfully cope with their illnesses, accomplish their recovery goals and excel toward the futures of their choice.

THERE IS NO LIFE WITHOUT MENTAL HEALTH

Obtaining and maintain their survival skills in the face of tragedies, is a reward to be viewed as strengths, not as weaknesses. They are also necessary tools for the day-to-day survival of mental illness.

THEIR OPTIMISM WAS BASED ON THE HOPE OF A POSITIVE, PROMISING FUTURE.

IMPORTANT COPING TIPS MY DAUGHTER LEARNED DURING THEIR JOURNEYS

☐ Never, ever look back.

☐ Take one day at a time; enjoy the good days and do not worry about the days that are disappointing or challenging.

☐ Display empathy and support toward each other.

☐ Learn long-suffering, kindness, and be self-sacrificing.

☐ Cling to hope.

☐ Find strength and courage.

☐ Be determined.

Clinging to Hope

How can this be happening again?" I kept repeating between my tears. My daughter was having a breakdown and I cannot do anything to stop it.

She was the sweetest young girl and I was proud of her. She was kind, caring and loved everyone. During the first six years of my son's illness, she supported and comforted me. She was my rock. She spent countless days by my side when I was sad and in anguish. **She cried when I cried.** She was my perfect, caring daughter.

Preparation and awareness were two key elements that helped me with preventing ANY relapses.

It was of paramount importance to me to have full confidence in my daughter's ability to heal. My confidence in her abilities strengthened her and made it easier for her to keep trying. She needed reassurance more than ever during this frightening time.

However, those challenges and obstacles were paving the way to coping, as more tragedies were yet to come. We would now be faced with the challenge of coping with the deaths of many loved ones.

Attitudes That Helped Her Cope

Following, is a list of the attitudes that helped my daughter to begin recovering:

☐ *She accepted their illnesses.*

☐ *She personally decided to begin their recovery journey.*

☐ *She was ready and willing to make lifestyle changes that bridged to her specific roads to recovery.*

☐ *She understood and accepted that, although there is no cure for mental illness, there is hope for living a quality life within the established economic system.*

☐ *She understood that the required journey required her to take one-step at a time.*

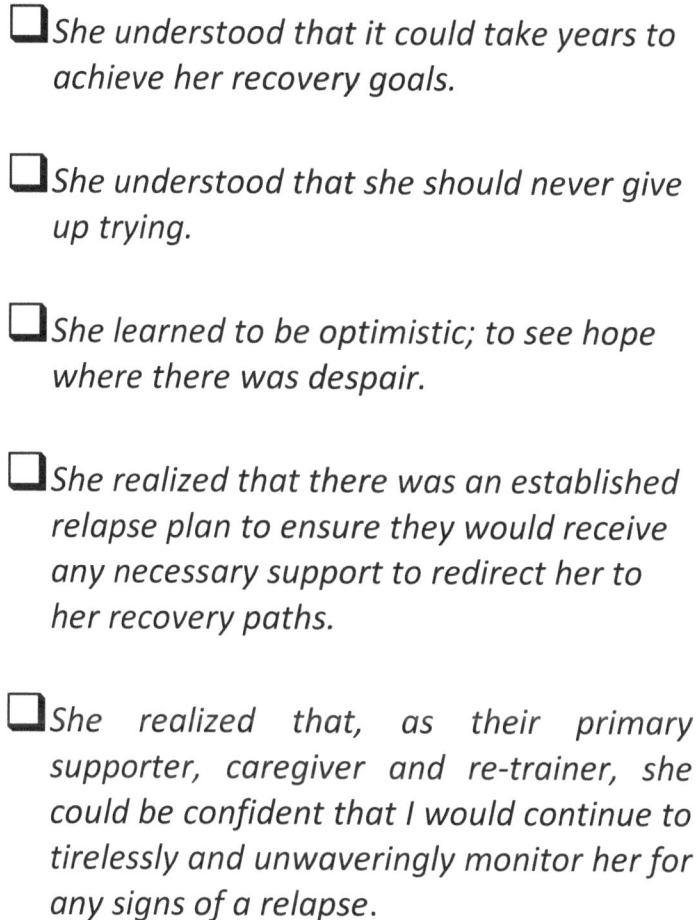

☐ *She understood that it could take years to achieve her recovery goals.*

☐ *She understood that she should never give up trying.*

☐ *She learned to be optimistic; to see hope where there was despair.*

☐ *She realized that there was an established relapse plan to ensure they would receive any necessary support to redirect her to her recovery paths.*

☐ *She realized that, as their primary supporter, caregiver and re-trainer, she could be confident that I would continue to tirelessly and unwaveringly monitor her for any signs of a relapse.*

The healing process also involved taking her antipsychotic medications as scheduled and at the correct dosage, in addition to being the recipients of love, care, on-going support, respect, understanding and allowing her to make her recovery time-frame her own. These ingredients were the central components of her healing.

The recovery process was frustrating, but by taking one-step-at-a-time, she improved a little each day.

In the end, her personal interpretation of how she felt determined her recovery progress. She is the only one that can say with certainty that she has recovered.

Attitudes that helped my daughter in her healing process are as follows:

☐ She accepted her illness.

☐ She had a clear vision of recovery.

☐ She believed that her recovery was possible.

☐ She had the desire to recover.

☐ She had a strong Will to work towards recovery.

☐ She stayed focused.

☐ She was positive.

☐ She received the proper medications and the correct dosages.

☐ She had unconditional family love, care, support, understanding and a strong nuclear-family support system.

☐ She knew her limitations and accepted them.

☐ She was persistent in finding ways to cope.

☐ She took one-step at a time.

☐ She looked at the bright side of life.

☐ She took a positive view of her illnesses.

☐ She had a positive view of the future.

☐ She found compassionate and supportive friends.

☐ She found neighbors who were encouraging and reassuring.

☐ She focused on what she could do instead of worrying about what she could not do.

☐ She kept she hope alive, and never wavered.

☐ She exercised regularly: walking, swimming and playing basketball.

☐ She had a stable routine: balanced diet and plenty of sleep.

☐ She engaged in regular, positive and worthwhile fun activities.

☐ She displayed strength, courage, determination, persistence and strength in the face of adversities.

☐ She had a daily household routine.

☐ She talked about her illnesses.

❏ She focused on developing healthy habits.

❏ She read success stories about people recovering from mental illnesses.

❏ She visited sick friends in their homes, the hospitals and nursing homes.

❏ She encouraged friends who were discouraged.

❏ Most of all she was hopeful of a bright future.

These attitudes have been instrumental in helping my daughter to progress. By combining my training with these attitudes, she developed the personal skills as well as job readiness skills that have resulted in enjoyment of her fulltime job and her optimism for the future.

Simple Fun Things the Family Enjoyed

For the first several years, amidst my daughter's bleakest periods, from the beautiful coastlines of Southern California to the awesome Blue Ridge Mountains in North Carolina, we enjoyed many fun, simple activities that were free, but effective in helping my family to cope with the mental illnesses. Besides prescribed medication, therapy and my unconditional love, below is a list of the fun and simple activities that we enjoyed and that helped in the coping and recovery process:

❏ Days when my daughter felt like walking helped a lot. We took long walks and enjoyed the fresh air.

❏ On lovely, beautiful, sunny days, we loved walking in the sunshine.

❏ We sun tanned to a golden brown along with our daily exercise.

❏ The fresh smell and the dramatic beauty of the flowers and blooming trees helped us enjoyed the day even more.

☐ Strolling around town on cool, breezy days was refreshing.

☐ Walks under beautiful moonlit skies and bright starry nights were very calming.

☐ Feeding the birds and watched them, which filled us with a feeling of freedom.

☐ Went walking on many nature trails and enjoyed the openness of the outdoors.

☐ We strolled around ponds and fed ducks.

☐ There were countless days spent relaxing in beautiful parks, enjoyed delicious picnic lunches and ate fresh berries and ripe watermelons.

☐ We reclined in the lush, green grass and read, and studied the bible. Other times we just meditated.

☐ On good days, we spent countless hours playing tennis and basketball.

☐ We spent many hours walking on sandy beaches and enjoyed the cool ocean breeze. We watched the elegant surfers. We went looking for unusual seashells. We enjoyed many picnic lunches, enjoyed many bon fires on cool nights and ate marshmallows straight from the fire pits. We enjoyed sharing our food with the birds that always seemed hungry!

☐ We enjoyed hiking up trails to the many wonderful waterfalls, and relaxed in the cool, refreshing waters of the Blue Ridge Mountains in Western North Carolina.

☐ On cool, breezy days, we took leisurely, daily walks to the local library and read many books that really interested us.

☐ Our small town main street helped us. We enjoyed many relaxing walks on downtown Main Street, ate ice cream cones and enjoyed delicious pastries.

☐ The local mall was a hangout place for us. We walked and window-shopped at local malls and enjoyed eating an egg roll or two.

☐ Calmness was important. We listened to calming music such as beautiful religious melodies. We also enjoyed listening to a wide variety of tranquility music.

❑ Water was calming for us. We swam at the pool, lounged under the sun or enjoyed a picnic lunch. Other times we just relaxed in the Jacuzzi.

❑ Exercise was important to us; and we frequently worked out at the gym.

❑ On weekends, we enjoyed friendly, home-based and park gatherings.

❑ We loved and enjoyed watching old movies.

❑ My daughter and I especially enjoyed massages and chiropractic treatments. Both helped to reduce our emotional pain and stress.

❑ We loved gardening. During the summer, we spent countless hours mowing the lawn and planted beautiful flowers. My daughter and I spent countless hours in Lowe and Home Depot home gardening stores.

❑ Many times, we relaxed at fast food eateries such as Arby's, McDonalds, Burger King, Kentucky Fried Chicken, and we especially enjoyed Long John Silver from time to time. Since we were on a tight budget, we took advantage of buy one get one free coupons from mailings and occasionally from the back of grocery store receipts. These were fun times that afforded us the opportunity to build a strong relationship and a stronger bond with each other.

☐ Continuous reinforcement of our family bonds by spending as much time as possible enjoying each other and developing their skills for the workforce.

Her Recovery Process

My daughter is still recovering from her illness. Although there is no known cure, there are effective medicines that control some of the symptoms of bipolar.

Recovery was long, difficult and frustrating. At first, it was almost impossible to access that road. Continuing was even more difficult, as it was bumpy with twists and turns along steep, narrow, sudden curves that, if not skillfully navigated, would have most definitely resulted in plummeting into deep ravines from which there was no rescue. Many times, giving up seem easier.

It has been stated that people with bipolar mood disorders have high mortality rates ranging from 35% higher to twice as high as the general population.

In spite of the grimness and hopelessness of the situation, my daughter found paths to endurance and perseverance, which spurred her to continue her recovery journey.

There were numerous obstacles to her recovery. All along the way, there were obstacles. There were many periods of highs and lows; positives and negatives. There were smiles and laughter, as well as sadness and tears. We enjoyed many joyous times as well as much sadness. There were challenges, fears, stressors and depression. In light of these, we quickly realized that it would take a one day at a time approach to begin her recovery process.

How she viewed her life situation was central to her recovery process.

My passion and drive for her recovery was foremost in my mind, and that propelled me to continue using my skills to encourage and support her.

Was recovery possible for my daughter?

ABSOLUTELY!

Yes, even though her recovery was slow she understood that the path to recovery was not the same for any two individuals. While she experienced many severe relapses, she progressed toward recovery at her own pace.

My daughter's last relapse was several years ago. Recovery is an on-going process for her. Her willingness to begin recovering required great courage and individual self-commitment to access her paths to recovery. Her decisions to begin recovering inspired me.

Her Progress

The most significant achievement of my daughter's recovery process was her acceptance of responsibility for managing her mental health care. My greatest joy is sharing in her experiences of unparalleled success to the point that I can safely use the term, "recovering." I am convinced that it was -- and continues to be -- her self-commitment, desire for well-being and overall optimism that, combined with my devotion and practical skills development training, has resulted in putting her on her road to recovery.

Even though my daughter has struggled throughout a significant portion of the last 17 years, she has worked tirelessly at stabilizing her illness. She applied the techniques in the Workbooks that I wrote, and is employed fulltime.

Today, her outlook on life is bright and promising. She is now optimistic that she will, one day, experience her dream of marriage and family.

I applaud my daughter for all their efforts. Their progress surpasses my expectations. I am amazed at how well they are progressing.

The resiliency she displayed is **OUTSTANDING**! Her progress to date is **REMARKABLE**!

Today, I am inspired to share my journey with everyone.

Today, I know that managing mental illness and being a contributing member of society is possible.

Today, I am inspired to share my coping and recovery empowerment methods and job training skills with others who want to access their path to recovery.

Epilogue

Thank you very much for reading this book and sharing my daughter's journey with me. When my son and daughter journeys with mental illness first began over two decades ago, I did not know when it would end or if it would ever end.

All four of my children were healthy children, so I had no concerns that one-day mental illness would become the center of my family's lives. One is never ready for this kind of illness!

In looking back now, I can see how ignorant and naive I had been about mental illness, and for that my daughter as well as the entire family paid a very high price.

From the inception of her bipolar, I knew that my daughter would need my fulltime support. Without hesitancy or any reservations and with the experience and skills I gained in caring for my son who is suffering with schizophrenia, I armed myself with that knowledge I had and took on this most unique and difficult assignment. I maintained my strength and courage.

My work took me on a life's journey that I could not have ever imagined.

My patience and skills in caring for both my son and daughter was necessary to the fullest degree. The job required strength, endurance, dedication and self-control beyond anyone's imagination.

The successes that I had achieved in taking charge of this illness were dependent upon my willingness to put all my efforts into this work.

Every family experiences periods of storminess in their lives. There are storms that leave very little damage, and storms that are devastating. The latter storms sweep away one's life. How each of us handles the clean up after those storms, determines how well each person will survive and rebuild his/her lives.

That is why it is important for parents and families to take charge and know the symptoms of schizophrenia and bi-polar disorders, as well as other mental illnesses and disorders.

My deck of cards that life gave me afforded me the opportunity to show kindness to others and to shine as a caring person.

Giving my daughter emotional support during the recovery process was important. Empowering her and motivating her to recovery, was worth sacrificing my hopes, dreams and aspirations, and successes that I would have pursued. It gave me great joy, happiness, and a good feeling that I did something worthwhile for her.

My daughter needed to be empowered, and I was able to provide her with some of the tools for success. She has rebuilt her self-worth and continued her development. I have prepared her with soft skills training for life and for the workforce.

My life, was once lost in the gloom of my 'storms of life.' Today my life is now bright and hopeful because I do not dwell on my children's illnesses; I dwell on their courage. My children's strength was outstanding and I applaud them for their strength and courage under such difficult circumstances.

In reflecting on my long, arduous journey, I am pleased that I have devoted all my efforts and talents to helping my son and daughter with their journeys.

My journey was an almost impossible situation, but with courage, strength, determination, and endurance I won the fight against all odds.

The greatest legacy I will leave all of my children is to face adversities with courage, strength and NEVER LET GO OF HOPE.

Yes, there is much comfort in one United States Senator's hopeful and encouraging words, **"Our hope lies in a better tomorrow, in hopes that when the sunrises, and the dawn of day comes, it will shed more light into the cause, and perhaps someday a cure for mental illness!"**

Conclusion

Bipolar disorders affect over 24 million people worldwide. Bi-polar affects over 5 million in the United States. Millions of people around the globe are undiagnosed and left untreated. To date there is no cure for bipolar disorders.

It was a frustrating and challenging journey, but my daughter learned how to control the symptoms and how to live with this horrific illness. There are effective medicines available and taking her prescribed medications is the only thing that works best for her.

Parents all over America living in households and communities that create modern stressors should be concerned and worried about their children's mental health, keeping in mind that stress is an inducer of mental illness, especially if there are genetic predispositions to this neurological imbalance.

The reason for concern is that anyone's daughter or daughter, brother or sister, mother or father, friend acquaintance or neighbor could at any time succumbed to a neurological imbalance induced by daily stressors. It shatters lives and may take years to stabilize or result in never being able to return to a quality of life conducive to community living.

Coping is difficult. Accessing the road to recovery is even harder. To cope with mental illnesses, many may turn to illegal drugs, alcohol, or promiscuity in desperation to escape their feelings of bewilderment about what is happening to them.

Most may have feelings of hopelessness, uncertainty and despair. Many family relationships are broken, and marriages may fail. Too many may even turn to violence and crime, and instead of receiving the therapies and medication that they need, become housed in an already overcrowded and financially overburdened prison system.

The most unfortunate, who cannot cope, MAY COMMIT SUICIDE OR MURDER.

AMERICANS HAVE THE POWER TO CHANGE THESE OUTCOMES!

Studies have shown that mental illnesses lead to unemployment; homelessness; poverty; overcrowded street corners, parks;, jails and prisons systems; and increase overall criminal activity including white-collar crime, and violence in all its forms which is perpetrated onto healthy members of society in the form of domestic abuse, sexual harassment, sexual trafficking and child exploitation. If a person does not have access to the proper medical attention, left undiagnosed and untreated, a person will become despondent, and ultimately, may take his or her life, or endanger someone else's life. This is PROFOUNDLY DANGEROUS to a civil society and will result in its destruction one person at a time, one household at a time, one community at a time.

Thousands of the mentally ill are homeless. Studies have shown that, "At any given time, there are many more Americans with untreated severe psychiatric illnesses living on America's streets than are receiving care in hospitals. Americans with untreated schizophrenia and manic-depressive illness comprise one-third or 250,000, of the estimated 744,000 homeless population. The quality of life for these individuals is abysmal. Many are victimized regularly."

It has been stated that women with schizophrenia and bi-polar disorders are more likely to be raped multiple times.

It has been stated that adequate mental health care is lacking in ALL American cities. It continues to be a problem, and is associated with high levels of social burden and cost partially leading to municipal financial failure, as well as an incalculable amount of individual pain and suffering.

From my daughter's shocking diagnosis and a disheartening prognosis of practically '**no hope of recovery**,' to glimmers of hope of recovery, then on to the recovering period. This progress has encouraged me to write this book to promote a mentally healthy America one person at a time, one family at a time, one community at a time, one city at a time.

The pain from bi-polar is real. Her pain was real. I kept reassuring her that she will get well again.

My children had no control over their mental disorders, so I made sure that I never blamed them for anything they did because of their illnesses. Blaming a person because of mental illness is cruel. It makes them feel even more depressed.

Viewing bipolar as a serious sickness rather than a weakness will help us focus on how we can support our loved one.

Quotations

"Bipolar affective disorder – This disorder affects about 60 million people worldwide. It typically consists of both manic and depressive episodes separated by periods of normal mood. Manic episodes involve elevated or irritable mood, over-activity, …. Decreased need for sleep, inflated self-esteem," stated the World Health Organization 2014.

"Bipolar disorder also known as manic-depressive disorder is a condition characterized by depressive episodes interspersed with periods of which mood and energy are excessively elevated well beyond normal levels of a good mood," stated **Barbara D. Ingersoll and Sam Goldstein**.

"Bipolar disorders affected 60 million people globally. In the United States, bipolar disorder affect 2 percent of the population," **World Health Organization (2014.)**

"Isolation was behind the recent surge in suicides by middle-aged men in Japan," stated **Kenshiro Ohara, a psychiatrist at Hamamatsu University School of Medicine in Japan.**

"Bipolar is a phantom that can sneak up on its victim cloaked in the darkness of melancholy but they disappear for years at a time only to return in the resplendent but fiery robes of mania," stated **Dr. Francis Mark Mondimore of the Johns Hopkins University School of Medicine.**

It has been stated that approximately 20% of children and adolescents experience mental disorders. Half of all mental illnesses begin by the age of 14. If untreated, these conditions severely influences children's development, their educational attainments and their potential to live fulfilling and productive lives.

"Bipolar is a phantom that can sneak up on its victim cloaked in the darkness of melancholy but the disappear for years at a time only to return in the resplendent but fiery robes of mania," stated Dr. Francis Mark Mondimore of the Johns Hopkins University School of Medicine.

"Traits of this illness include severe mood swings that vacillate between depression an mania. During the depressed phase, you may be haunted by thoughts of suicide. During the manic phase of the illness, your good judgment may evaporate and you may not be able to see the harm of your actions," – American Medical Association.

The National Mental Health Association stated**,** *"Mental health problems affect one in every five young people at any given time. An estimated two-thirds of all young people with mental health problems are not receiving the help they need."* The article further states, *"Suicide is the third leading cause of death for 15- to 24-years-olds and the sixth leading cause of death for 5- to 15-year-olds."*

It has been stated that people with bipolar mood disorders have high mortality rates ranging from 35% higher to twice as high as the general population.

According to Dr. Cheryl Lane, PhD. www.schizophrenia.com, *"Attempting to find new work after a diagnosis of schizophrenia can be particularly difficult. If a potential employer is aware of the person's diagnosis, discrimination may hinder landing a job. Also, significant stigma is associated with any major mental illness."*

"During the depressed phase, you may be haunted by thoughts of suicide. During the manic phase of the illness, your good judgment may evaporate and you may not be able to see the harm of your actions," – **American Medical Association.**

Dr. Lane further states, *"A possible solution for many individuals is to become involved in some sort of vocational training or rehabilitation program. They can learn new skills and get help with learning or improving social skills. These programs can also help them function more fully and develop better thinking skills. Additionally, working with a psychotherapist can help with self-esteem issues, stress management and making the best choices in terms of whether to work."*

Columbia University's Department of Psychiatry stated that *"To understand and promote recovery from serious mental illnesses, it is important to study the perspectives of individuals who are coping with mental health problems. The aim of the present study was to examine identity-related themes in published self-narratives of family members and individuals with serious mental illness. It adds to the body of* *research addressing how identity affects the process of recovery and identifies potential opportunities for using published narratives to support individuals as they move toward positive identities that facilitate recovery."*

The National Institute of Mental Health (NIMH), stated, *"Schizophrenia is a chronic, severe, and disabling brain disorder that has affected people throughout history. About 1 percent of Americans have the disease."*

World Fellowship for Schizophrenia and Allied Disorders, states, *"Schizophrenia is the most persistent and disabling of the major mental illness…While it is treatable in many cases there is yet no cure…"*

A psychiatrist, as recorded in a medical journal [16 (2) 2003], was quoted as saying, *"It is well known that schizophrenia is a chronic, generally life-long, mental illness that significantly debilitates afflicted individuals and severely compromises their function and quality of life."*

The Nutritional Management of Schizophrenia described schizophrenia in this way, *"Schizophrenia may be caused by genetic* *predisposing factors or environmental influences."*

University of Alberta Press Release, stated, *"Schizophrenia is a biochemical brain disorder characterized by delusions, disordered, thinking, hallucinations and a lack of motivation and energy."*

U.S. National Institutes of Mental Health (NIMH) stated**,** *"1.1 percent of the U.S. population age 18 and older in any given year."* *The article goes on to state, "Scientists have long known that Schizophrenia runs in families, it occurs in 10% of people who have first-degree relatives with the disorder." Additionally, it stated, "Many people with Schizophrenia improve enough to lead independent, satisfying lives."*

National Alliance on Mental Illness stated, *"Schizophrenia is a serious mental illness that affects 2.4 million American adults over the age of 18."*

The American Psychiatric Association stated regarding one possible cause of Schizophrenia, *"Although the origin of Schizophrenia has not been identified, Scientists know that there are* *some hereditary or genetic predispositions for the disease because it runs in families."*

American Psychiatric Association, Jeffrey Draine, Ph.D. and several or his colleagues wrote an article stated, *"With an improved understanding of the disease and effective therapies, those with schizophrenia can have a full life, hold a job, and live in the community or with their family."*

World Health Organization stated, *"More than 90% of all cases of suicide are associated with mental disorders such as depression, schizophrenia, and alcoholism,"* notes Dr. Benedetto Saraceno, Director of the Department of Mental Health for WHO, October 9, 2006.

The National Advisory Mental Health Council of the WHO stated, *"Schizophrenia is a (mental) disorder associated with high levels of social burden and cost, as well as an incalculable amount of individual pain and suffering."*

World Health Organization, *i*n a 1992 article, *quoted Leete as saying, "Stigma is shameful and displays a shameful part in human behavior. Stigma is damaging and destructive, it is a multi-layered and complex problem."*

WHO published an article by Deegan in 1980. *The article stated, "Stigmas act as a powerful barrier to treatment not because of the fear of being labeled as mentally ill, but because too often mental health professionals and mental health services as a whole, often in a subtle way display negative or rejecting attitudes towards users and perpetuate practices fostering segregation, dependency and powerlessness.*

The Queensland Alliance for Mental Health observed, "P*eople with mental health problems are "frequently the object of ridicule or derision and are depicted within the media as being violent, impulsive and incompetent." It also found that the myth surrounding violence has not been dispelled, despite evidence to the contrary.*

Mental Illness Policy stated, *"Americans with untreated schizophrenia and manic-depressive illness comprise one-third or 250,000, of the estimated 744,000 homeless population." The quality of life for these individuals is abysmal. Many are victimized regularly.* (mentalillnesspolicy.org)

Social Psychiatry and Psychiatric, in a 1994 study stated, *"Women with schizophrenia and bi-polar* *disorders are more likely to be raped multiple times."*

"People with bipolar mood disorders have high mortality rates ranging from 35% higher to twice as high as the general population. There is a 1.8 times higher risk of dying associated with depression. People with severe mental illness do not receive the same quality of physical health care as the general population," (WHO) 2015.

Resources

Depression and Bipolar Support Alliance (DBSA)
730 N. Franklin Street, Suite 501
Chicago, IL 60610-7204
Phone Number: (312) 642-0049
Toll-Free Number: (800) 826-3632
Fax Number: (312) 642-7243
www.dbsalliance.org

American Psychiatric Association
1000 Wilshire Blvd, Suite 1825
Arlington, VA 22209-3901
Phone Number: (703) 907-7300
Email Address: apa@psych.org
www.psych.org

World Health Organization
www.who.org

American Medical Association
www.ama.org

Author

Alyse King is the mother of four courageous children, one wonderful daughter and three delightful daughters. She is also a grandmother of one beautiful granddaughter and four adorable granddaughters.

For over two decades, Ms. King has tirelessly focused her attention on caring for two of her four children who had been struggling with chronic mental illnesses since they were teenagers. She has successfully helped them cope with their illnesses and reintegrate into society by retraining them to live independently and become financially self-reliant, provided them with the essential skills training that are vitally important to self-improvement and skills for the job market.

Ms. King's happiness about her ability to help her son and daughter has encouraged her to share the "recovery techniques" she used. She self-published eight books titled, "A Letter to Schizophrenia from a Mother," "Schizophrenia," "Bi-Polar," "Stress and Depression," "140 Ways

Coping with Depression," "Schizophrenia, Bi-Polar, Stress and Stigmas," "Finding Hope in a Hopeless World," and a self-help Workbook titled, "Day After Day Coping with Mental Illness - Support for Individuals and Families."

Alyse King also self-published one Trainers' Guide and three Self-Help Guides titled, "Reintegrating after Traumatic Life Experience for: "Self Improvement," "Job Preparation," and "How to Keep Your Job." The Workbooks provide continuing education and training for returning to employment or becoming financially independent. The Workbooks share the systematic techniques that Ms. King used in helping her children to develop personal skills and skills for hunting for a job, securing the job and holding the job.

The Trainers' Manual provides guidance to all who wish to develop programs to help others to find work or achieve financial independence.

Alyse also self-published four other books, "Comfort and Hope – Death- Reflections from Scriptures," "A 30-Day Online Romance, Based on a True Story - Part 1," "Confessions from A 30-Day Online Romance, Based on a True Story - Part 2, and "A Follow-Up of Confessions from A

30-Day Online Romance, Based on a True Story - Part 3."

Ms. King grew up and was educated on a beautiful Caribbean Island; married in her 20's and has been a homemaker, mother and sole provider for her family. Later, divorced, she relocated to Southern California with her four children.

The author currently resides in the beautiful Blue Ridge Mountains in Western North Carolina. Her daughter and youngest daughter also live in North Carolina. Her other two eldest daughters and all five grandchildren remain in Southern California. She frequently travels to California to visit her family and friends.

Ms. King's goal is to utilize her expertise in both the health and educational sectors. For the past several years, she has been working towards that goal by volunteering her time to help friends who are struggling to cope with mental illness.

Website: cmitrainingservices.com
E-mail: cmitrainingservices@gmail.com
http://www.amazon.com/-/e/B001KE71BQ
https://www.smashwords.com/books/search?query=alyse+king

http://www.linkedin.com/in/alyseking
https://www.facebook.com/alyse.king.12382

NOTES

NOTES

www.ingramcontent.com/pod-product-compliance
Lightning Source LLC
Chambersburg PA
CBHW070822180526
45168CB00002B/728